MW00785243

# Stretch Your Stress Away with ShaNay

LAEL PUBLISHING

STRETCH YOUR STRESS AWAY WITH SHANAY
A Guide To A More Flexible And Relaxed You
by ShaNay Norvell
Published by The Lael Agency
Winston Salem, North Carolina
www.LaelAgency.com

No part of this book may be used or reproduced in any form, stored in a retrieval system, or transmitted in any form by any means, electronic, photocopy, mechanical, recording or otherwise without written permission from the author. The only exception is for critical articles or reviews, in which brief excerpts may be used.

Cover Photo: Donna Permell

Paperback ISBN - 978-1-7325344-6-9

Author's contact:
Email: ShaNay@ShaNayNorvell.com
Website: ShaNayNorvell.com

Copyright © 2019 by ShaNay Norvell

All Rights Reserved

First Edition

Printed in the United States of America.

# DEDICATION

I dedicate this book to my mother, who told me everything I touched turned to gold when I was a child.

I dedicate this book to my father, who has unwavering faith in me.

I would like to dedicate this book to my sister, who is really my third parent and has had my back since I came out of my mother's womb.

I would like to dedicate this book to my son Bakari to show you that you too can do whatever you want to do if you put your mind to it! You are my sunshine!

May my words, actions, and energy touch and heal the lives of others.

Thank you to my entire family and village.

Proceeds of this book go to Family Ties and other agencies and organizations that help heal victims of sexual abuse and domestic violence.

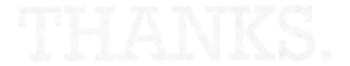

THANKS.

I would like to thank the following for their participation in the production of this book:

Photographer: Donna Permell
Make Up: Kiona Forston
Styling: Cherise B. Thomas

# CONTENTS

## Why Stretch?

You are a full energetic being. Energy is neither created nor destroyed, it merely moves to another location. Stretching your body moves energy from the top of your head to the soles of your feet.

There are many who believe yoga is the only way to stretch the body and gain more flexibility. It is not the only way. It is a way. Yoga historically has created an inner peace as well as a physical release. From a religious standpoint, it has been helpful to prepare for meditation.

But this is the story for many, but it may not be the story for you. You are on the go. Your schedule is busting at the seams and adding a yoga class is not an option. Religion may not be your thing. Your mind is too busy to meditate.

But I can tell you this: You have a moment to stretch. You have 10 minutes to stretch. You NEED to stretch.

## Why Do You Need to Stretch?

One word – STRESS.
Stress is ever present and can come from positive things or negative things. It can be....

- Planning for a wedding (Positive Source)
- Planning a funeral (Negative Source)
- College graduation (Positive Source)
- Divorce (Negative Source)
- Starting a new job (Positive Source)
- A newborn child (Positive Source)

No one can escape stress. However, we can all learn to embrace it and manage it appropriately. One of the greatest tools I have learned to use to manage stress is stretching.

**I will help you stretch the stress away.**

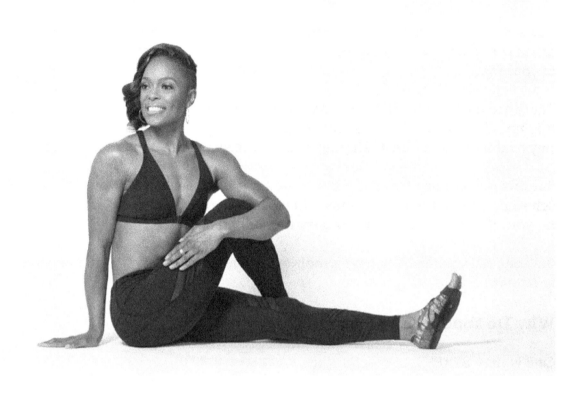

In this guide, you will learn how to move your body in ways that will release tension, lengthen your muscles, relax and energize you.

The movements are not extra, they are necessary to make the most of your stretching sessions.

In this guide I have combined my favorite Yoga, Pilates, and functional body movements to tailor this stretching program towards stress reduction, energy flow, and revitalization.

## What Does Stress Do to your Body?

When you are stressed, your body tightens. Your muscles prepare for flight or fight. Adrenaline is pumping and your heart is racing. Blood pressure increases. This can happen for a short period of time or over a longer period. Over time your muscles are getting tighter as more tension is building. You will begin to feel stiff. Your neck, shoulders, and lower back are usually the areas that start whispering to you in the form of tightness, tenderness, and tension.

For example, have you ever had anyone walk behind you and unexpectedly massage your shoulders? It is like heaven, or at least your idea of heaven. You close your eyes, your head drops, and you breathe a sigh of relief. You needed that. Your muscles needed that.

The other signs of stress from a physiological standpoint can manifest through tension headaches.

Over time what does stress and the tension it produces in our body do? It limits your range of motion. It shortens your stride. It can simply make you cranky. All these feelings and factors can be stretched away.

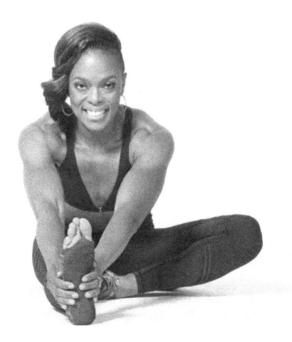

## Why Do You Need to Relax?

Relaxation and stretching go hand in hand. When you relax into your stretch, you will get more out of it. When you stretch properly, you will find your stress melts away and you become more relaxed.

Breathing deeply and completely is a key to relaxation. Putting your mind into a peaceful state will help you gain the maximum benefit, even from a short stretching session. Inhale deeply. As you exhale, imagine your body going deeper into the stretch, your muscles getting looser, your body getting more relaxed.

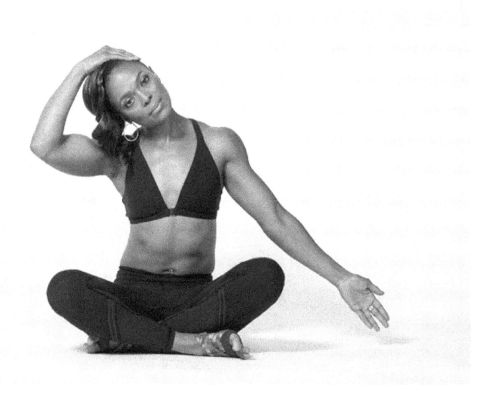

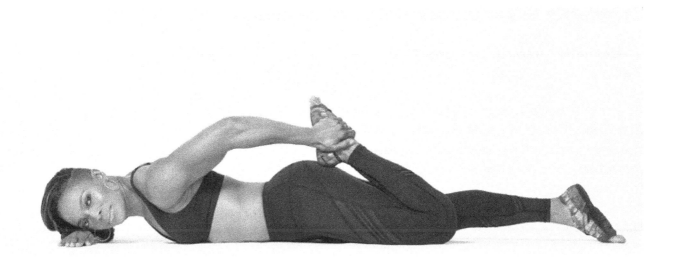

## Benefits of Stretching the Stress Away

1. You will feel less uneasy. You will feel the tension leave your body, replaced by feelings of lightness and ease.

2. You will gain more clarity and notice an increase in mental stimulation.

3. Blood flow is increased throughout the body, improving circulation.

4. Your body will produce happy hormones which gives you an endorphin high. This is the best natural high you can ask for. It can almost make you feel giddy, tranquil, and peaceful.

5. Better sleep will often follow, especially if you are able to stretch in the evening.

## Frequently Asked Questions About Stretching

**1. How often should you stretch?**
Daily.

**2. Do you need to warm up before stretching?**
Yes. The ideal scenario is that you have been moving your muscles prior to stretching. This is more important than temperature. However, although this will help you make the most of your stretching, it is not required.

There are preparatory movements you can do to help. See my video of one of my favorite martial arts movements.

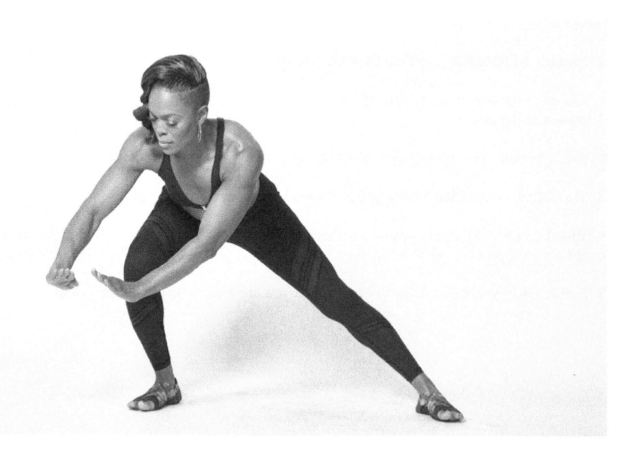

Stand with your legs just a little wider than shoulder width. Outstretch your hands, palms facing outwards. Imagine you are drawing a figure 8 or infinity sign in the sand on a beach, with your hands about two feet above the ground. Slowly drag your hands across the sand in a controlled motion. Bend your knees and glide side to side in a rhythmic motion.

### 3. How do I know how much pressure to use during the stretching?

When you first start a regular stretch routine, it may feel uncomfortable but should not feel painful. You want to stretch to a point of discomfort but not a point of pain. Listen to your body. When you feel the tension, or the muscle tighten release the stretch a little and hold. Then use your breathing to go deeper into the stretch or continue to hold. Also, be patient with the process. You want to incrementally increase the pressure and over time increase the range.

## Stretch with ShaNay

### Getting Started – What do you need?

You and your body are the main requirements. However, over the years I have worked with clients who have difficulty getting down on the floor and/or getting up from the floor. I have incorporated stretches that can be done while you are sitting. Be sure to grab a sturdy chair. You will see my demonstrations include a basic folding chair. These variations may also be useful for people new to stretching who may lack the flexibility of those who are more experienced with this practice.

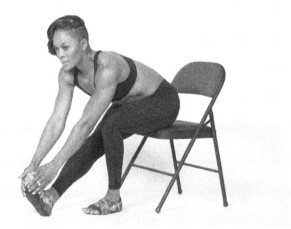

# STRETCHES.

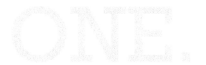

# Neck Stretch

Sit on the edge of a seat or couch, feet flat on the floor. Take a deep breath in. As you exhale, imagine a light thread touching the top of your head, extending to the sky. Take another deep breath in. As you exhale slowly, lean your right ear down to your right shoulder, without moving your torso. Hold this for 15 slow intentional counts. Breath in slowly and with control.

After you count to 15, take a deep breath in, and as you exhale, bring your head to the center. Inhale again, and as you exhale, lean your head toward your left ear. Hold 15 slow deliberate counts. Inhale and exhale, slowly bringing your head back to the center.

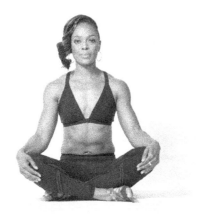
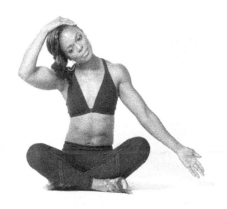

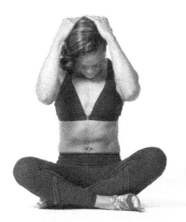
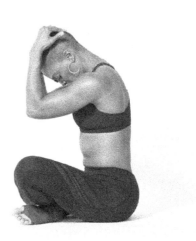

*Neck Stretch*

## 2.  Spine Stretch

Start seated with your legs both extended in front of you.  Cross your left leg over your right leg and try to place your left foot on the floor.  Extend your right arm up to the sky.  Twist your body toward your left leg.  Lower your right arm and place it behind your left leg on the floor. Inhale deeply.  As you exhale, twist your body deeper to the left.  Keep your gaze over your left shoulder...and smile. Hold 15 to 30 seconds. Repeat on the other side.

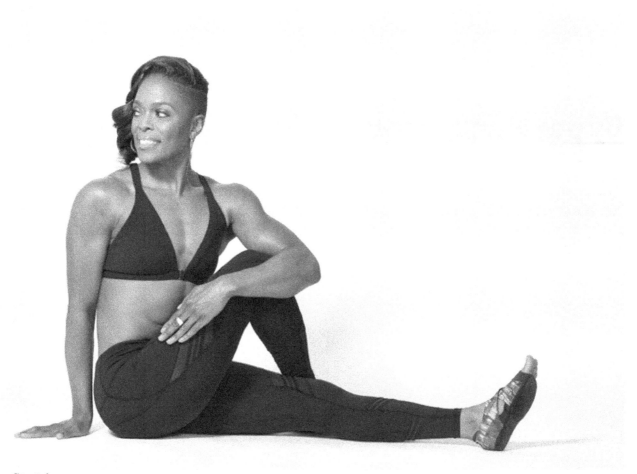

*Spine Stretch*

# THREE

# Upper Back Stretch

Start seated with your legs both extended in front of you. Extend both of your arms in front of you at shoulder level. Interlace your fingers, palms facing you. Inhale deeply. As you exhale, round out your upper back as if a ball was pressing against your chest. Hold 15 to 30 seconds, 3 rounds.

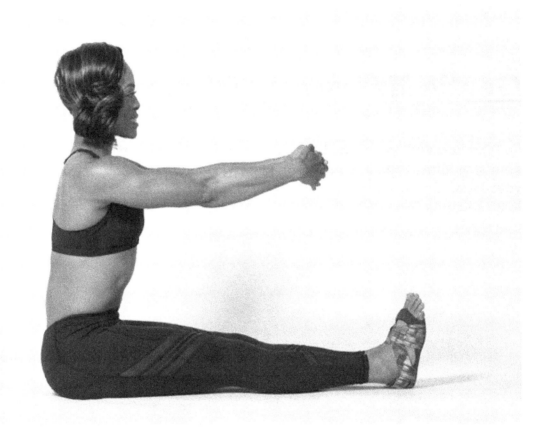

*Upper Back Stretch*

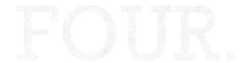FOUR.

# Gentle Hamstring Stretch

Start seated with your legs both extended in front of you. Place your hands on your thighs, knees, or shins. Inhale deeply. As you exhale slowly, lean forward sliding your hands down your legs. Once you feel resistance or tightening of your hamstrings, pull back and hold 15 to 30 seconds. Repeat 3 times.

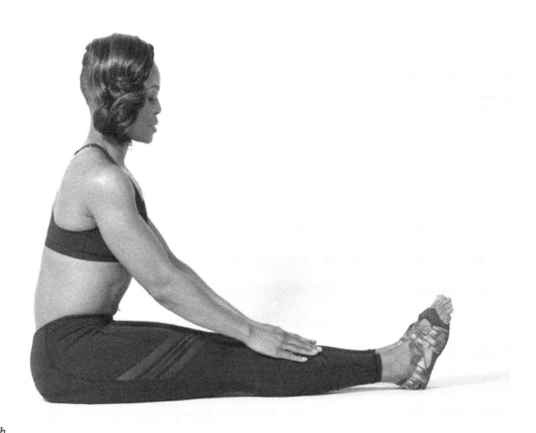

*Gentle Hamstring Stretch*

# FIVE

# Spine Lengthener Stretch

Start seated with your legs both extended in front of you. This stretch is similar to the gentle hamstring stretch. Place your hands on your thighs. Inhale deeply. As you exhale lean forward from lower back. Extend from your lower back to the crown of your head. Feel your spine lengthen. Inhale and continue to lean forward. As you exhale, extend from your spine, continuing the stretch through and to the crown of your head. Repeat 5 times.

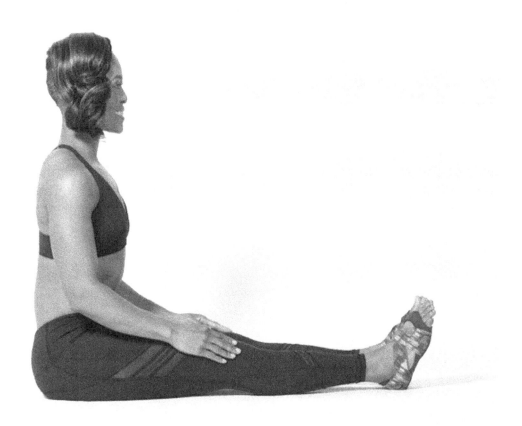

Spine Lengthener Stretch

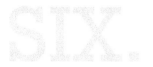

# Forward Spine Stretch

Start seated with your legs both extended in front of you. Extend your arms straight out in front of you shoulder level. Inhale deeply. As you exhale, lengthen through your spine and reach through your fingertips. Feel your shoulder blades spread out and open. Hold 15 seconds. Repeat 6 times.

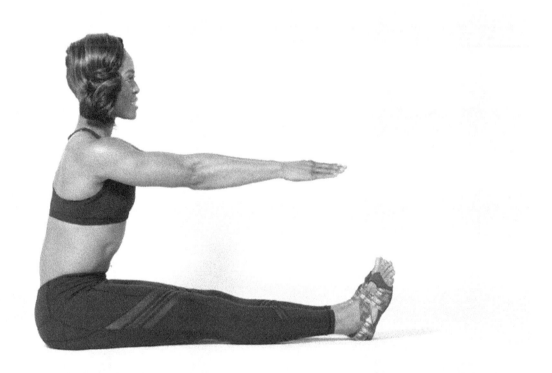

*Forward Spine Stretch*

# SEVEN

# Intermediate Hamstring Stretch

Start seated with your legs both extended in front of you. Draw your right leg in toward your groin and place your right foot alongside your knee. Place both hands on your left thigh. Inhale deeply. As you exhale slowly, lean forward and slide your hands down your left leg. Once you feel your hamstring tighten, pull back a few inches. Hold that position and inhale and exhale 15 seconds. Repeat 3 times on left leg then switch to other leg.

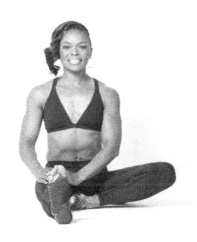

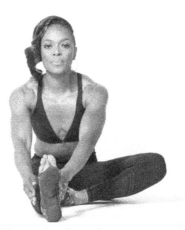

*Intermediate Hamstring Stretch*

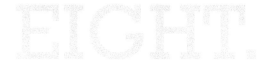

# Deepened Hamstring Stretch

This stretch is an advanced version of the intermediate hamstring stretch. Start seated with your legs both extended in front of you. Draw your right leg in toward your groin and place your right foot alongside your knee. Place both hands on your left knee. Inhale deeply. As you exhale slowly, lean forward and slide your hands down toward your left foot. Once you feel you hamstring tighten, pull back a few inches. Hold that position and inhale and exhale 30 seconds. Repeat 3 times on left leg then switch to other leg.

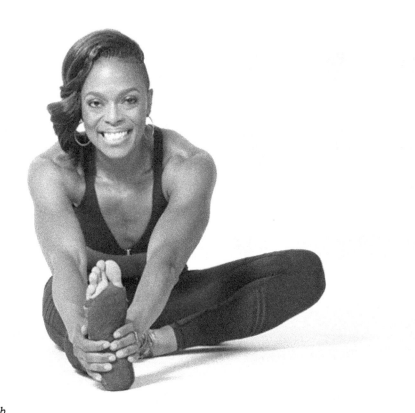

*Deepened Hamstring Stretch*

# Butterfly Stretch

Start seated with your legs both extended in front of you. Draw both of your legs in toward your groin and place the soles of your feet together. Hold your ankles and place your elbows on your inner thighs. Inhale deeply. As you exhale, press your elbows into your inner thighs. Hold 15 seconds. Release the pressure gently and flutter your legs. Repeat 4 times.

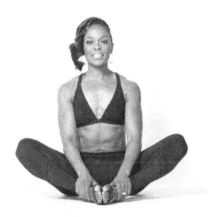
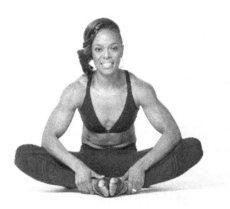
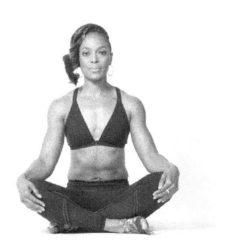

*Butterfly Stretch*

# TEN

# Wrist Tension Release Stretch

Sit comfortably on the floor with your legs crossed.  Extend your right arm out in front of you at shoulder level.  Point your fingers down toward the floor.  Hold your right hand with your left hand and gently press your right thumb into your palm. Hold 15 seconds. Repeat 2 times. Switch to other side.

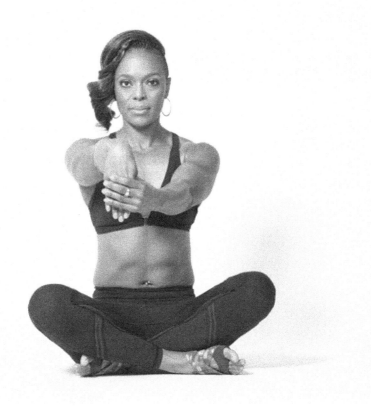

*Wrist Tension Release Stretch*

# ELEVEN

# Wrist Tension Extensor

Sit comfortably on the floor with your legs crossed. Extend your right arm out in front of you at shoulder level. Point your fingers up toward the ceiling. Hold your right hand with your left hand and gently press your right thumb into the back of your hand. Hold 15 seconds. Switch to the other side.

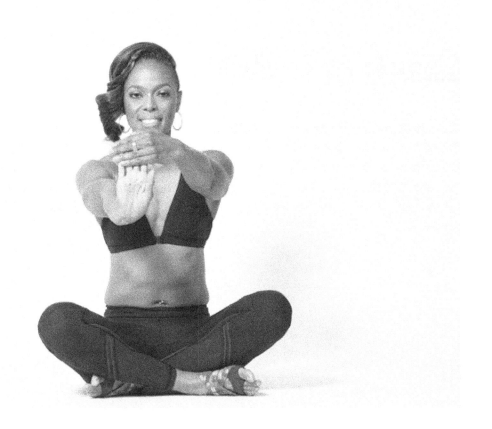

*Wrist Tension Extensor*

# TWELVE

# Shoulder Stretch

Sit comfortably on the floor with your legs crossed. Extend your right arm in front of you. Slowly take the right arm across your body. Place your left hand on your right arm between the elbow and the wrist. Firmly hold the right arm in your left hand. Inhale deeply. As you exhale gently, pull the right arm closer to your body. Keep your right shoulder down and away from your chin. Hold 15 seconds. Switch to the other arm. Repeat stretch on both arms 2 times.

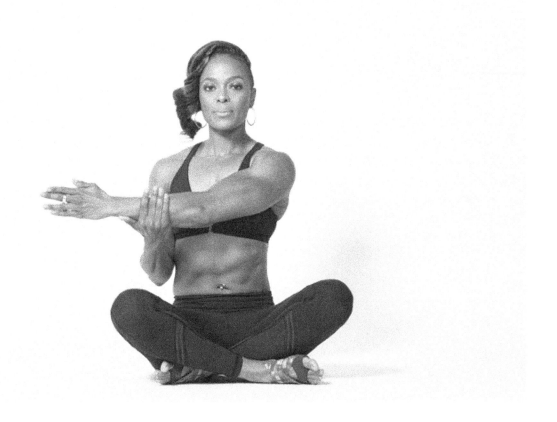

*Shoulder Stretch*

THIRTEEN.

# Tricep Stretch

Sit comfortably on the floor with your legs crossed. Extend your right arm up toward the sky with energy extending through your fingertips. Bend the right arm at the elbow and reach for your left shoulder with your right hand. Reach your left arm up and over placing your left hand on the side of your right elbow. Inhale deeply. As you exhale, gently place pressure on your right arm with you left hand. Hold this stretch for 15 seconds. Switch to the other arm. Repeat 2 times.

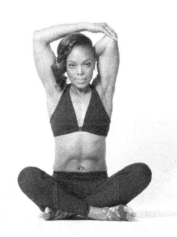

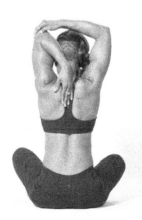

*Tricep Stretch*

# Inner Thigh and Groin Stretch

Start by placing your hands and your knees on the floor. Then slowly place your elbows on the floor. Inhale deeply. As you exhale, let your knees go out to the side feeling a stretch in your inner thigh and groin. Inhale deeply. As you exhale, relax your hips and lower back to give your body permission to go deeper into the stretch. Hold 20 to 30 seconds. Repeat 3 times.

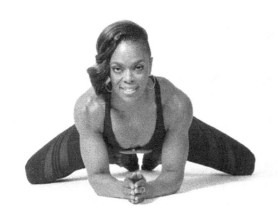

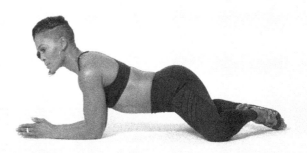

*Inner Thigh and Groin Stretch*

47

FIFTEEN

# Intense Hamstring Stretch

Start by lying on your back. Bend your right leg placing your right foot flat on the floor. Extend your left leg up toward the sky. Reach with both hands toward your thigh, calf, or ankle. Avoid placing your hands behind the knee. Inhale deeply. As you exhale, gently pull your left leg closer to your body. Inhale deeply. As you exhale, pull your leg closer to your body. Inhale deeply for a third time. As you exhale, pull your leg closer to your body slowly until you feel your hamstring resist or tighten. If you feel it tighten release it slowly and pause at a comfortable level. Now, hold that position for 25 to 30 seconds. Release and switch to the other leg. Repeat both legs 3 times.

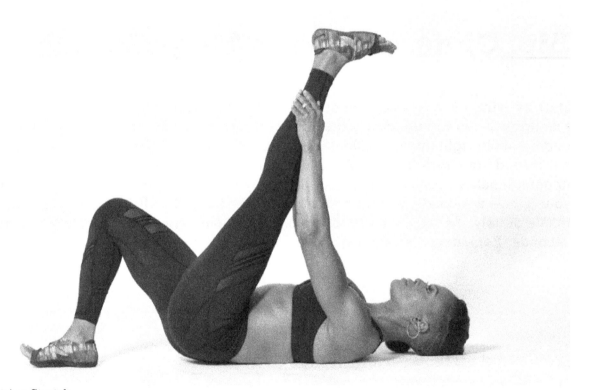

*Intense Hamstring Stretch*

# SIXTEEN

# Hip, Glute, and Outer Thigh Stretch

Start by lying on your back. Bend your right leg placing your right foot flat on the floor. Extend your left leg up toward the sky. Bend your left leg and place the left ankle on the middle of the right thigh. Inhale deeply. As you exhale, lift your head and reach both hands out toward your right thigh. Wrap your hands around your right thigh and interlace your fingers. Inhale deeply. As you exhale, extend your right leg toward the sky. Inhale deeply. As your exhale a second time lower your head to the floor. Slowly bend your left leg back down. Inhale deeply. As you exhale, gently pull the right leg closer to your body and hold 15 to 20 seconds. Repeat on both sides 2 times.

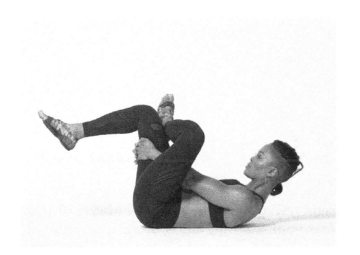
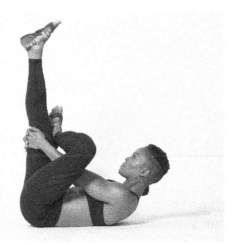

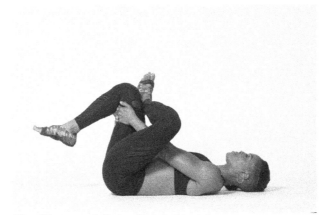

*Hip, Glute, and Outer Thigh Stretch*

# SEVENTEEN

# Low Back Compression Stretch

Start by lying on your back. Inhale deeply. Exhale and draw both your right leg and your left leg up to your chest. Take your right arm and your left arm across your legs and hug them gently at the knee. Inhale deeply. As you exhale, give yourself a firm hug pulling your knees deep into your body. Inhale deeply. As you exhale, keep the firm hug and hold for 20 seconds. Release both legs and repeat stretch again 2 times.

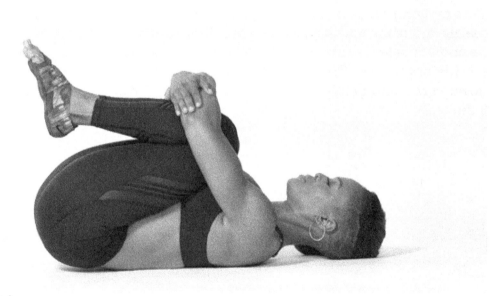

*Low Back Compression Stretch*

# EIGHTEEN

# Deep Inner Thigh & Low Back Stretch

Start by lying on your back. Inhale deeply. Draw both knees up toward your chest. As you exhale, touch the soles of your feet together and open your knees out to the side in a butterfly position. Inhale deeply. Exhale and lift your head up and reach your hands out to grab the outside of your feet. Try to interlace your fingers. Inhale deeply. Exhale and lower your head down to rest and gently pull your feet in closer to your groin. Hold 25 to 30 seconds. Repeat 3 times.

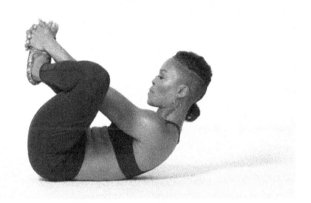

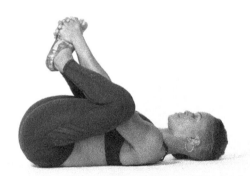

*Deep Inner Thigh and Low Back Stretch*

# NINETEEN

# Quadricep Stretch

Start by lying on your stomach. You can turn your face to the left and rest your head on your arm. Inhale deeply. Exhale and slowly bend your left leg at the knee. Extend your left arm back and gently hold your left leg at the ankle, pant leg, or heel of shoe. Inhale deeply. Exhale and continue to firmly hold your leg in bent position. Hold for 20 to 25 seconds. Repeat on both legs 2 times.

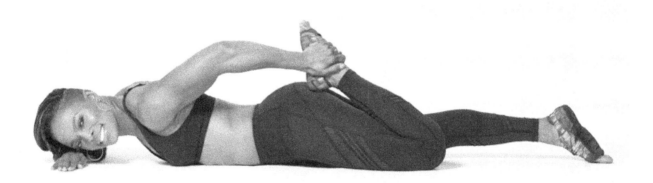

*Quadricep Stretch*

TWENTY.

# Advanced Quad and Hip Flexor Stretch

Start by kneeling on your left knee. Place right foot flat on the floor. Inhale deeply. Exhale and reach back toward your left leg lifting your left foot off the floor. Gently grab your left leg at the ankle, pant leg, or heel of your shoe. Inhale deeply. Exhale and hold for 20 seconds. Switch to other leg and repeat.

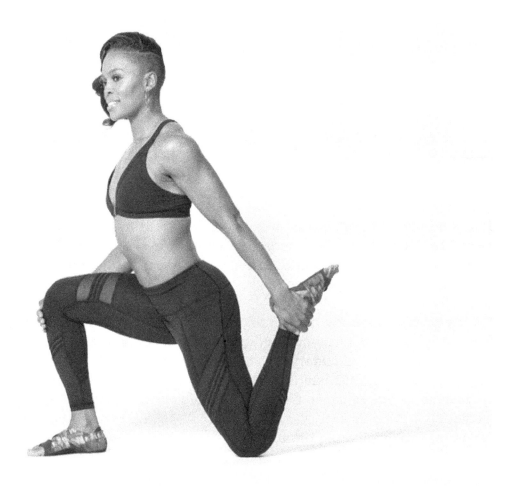

*Advanced Quad and Hip Flexor Stretch*

# TWENTY-ONE

# Inner Thigh Stretch Straddle

Start seated with legs separated in a straddle position. Place right hand on right thigh and left hand on left thigh. Inhale deeply. Exhale and relax the inner thigh muscles as much as possible. Now place both hands side by side on the floor in front of you. Inhale deeply. As you exhale, lean forward bending at the hips. Avoid lifting your knees. Inhale deeply. Exhale and lean forward deeper into the stretch. Hold for 25 seconds.

Slowly bring your body back to an upright position, sliding your hands back closer to your inner thighs. Now, turn your body to the right as well as your gaze. Place both hands on the right thigh. Inhale deeply. Exhale and lean forward bending at the hips. Inhale deeply. Exhale and slide your hands down toward your knee, shin, ankle, or foot. If you feel your hamstring, groin, or inner thigh tighten, slowly pull back. Once you are at a comfortable position, hold for 25 seconds. Slowly come back up to an upright position and repeat on the left side. Repeat all three parts 2 times.

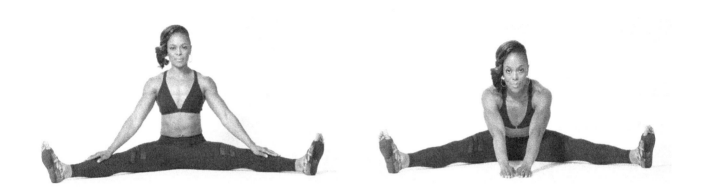

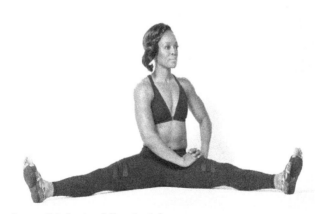

*Inner thigh straddle stretch*

# TWENTY-TWO

# Hip, Glute, and Outer Thigh Stretch Variation

Begin in a seated position with both legs extended in front of you. Draw your right leg in and place it on your left leg with your right ankle resting on your left thigh. Inhale deeply. Exhale and lean forward with the body toward your bent leg to deepen the stretch. You can also flex your left foot by lifting your toes off the floor. This will deepen the stretch. Inhale deeply. Exhale and hold 20 seconds. Repeat on both sides 2 times

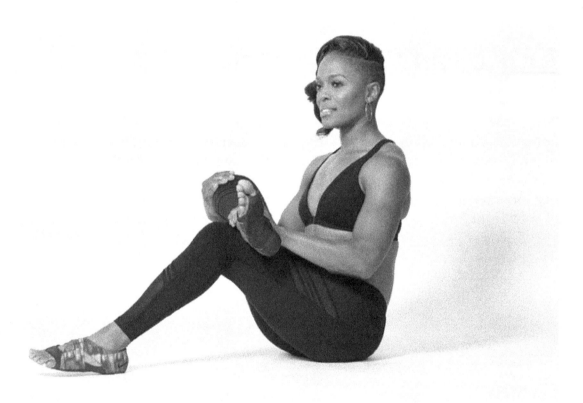

*Hip, Glute, and Outer Thigh Stretch Variation*

# Ankle Rotation Stretch

Begin this stretch in the position you ended the Hip, Glute, and Outer Thigh Stretch Variation. Begin in a seated position with both legs extended in front of you. Draw your right leg in and place it on your left leg with your right ankle resting your left thigh. Gently grab your right foot with your left hand. Inhale deeply. Exhale and slowly rotate the ankle of your right foot in a clockwise direction 5 times. Pause. Inhale deeply. Exhale and slowly rotate your ankle of your right foot in a counterclockwise direction 5 times. Switch sides and repeat.

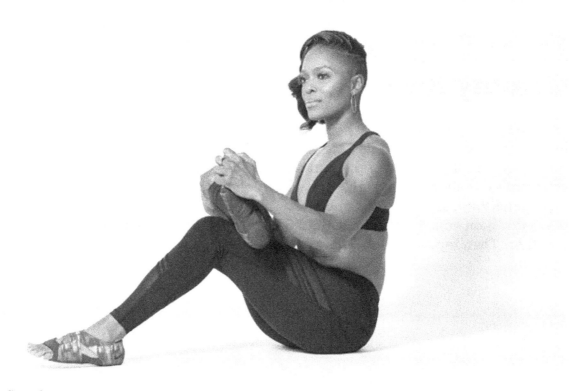

*Ankle Rotation Stretch*

# TWENTY-FOUR

# Inner Thigh Stretch Wall Variation Gravity Assist

Begin by lying on your back with your legs extending to the sky and your butt and heels resting on a wall. Inhale deeply. Exhale and slowly let your left leg slide to the left side and your right leg slide to the right. Inhale deeply. Exhale and place your right hand on your right inner thigh and your left hand on your left inner thigh. Inhale deeply. Exhale and gently press down on your inner thighs. Hold 30 seconds. Rest by slowly bringing your legs back together. Then repeat stretch 3 times.

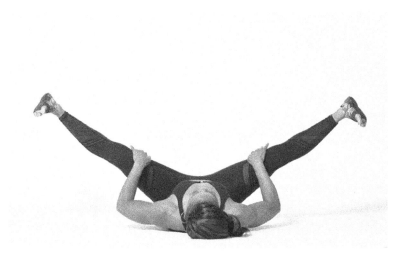

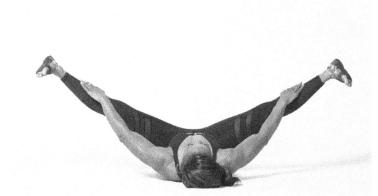

*Inner Thigh Stretch Wall Variation Gravity Assist*

67

TWENTY-FIVE.

# Spine Lengthener Variation Posture Check

When you stretch and exercise, your spine and vertebrae should lengthen and become stronger. It is important to be aware of your posture throughout the day. Keep your body lifted. Imagine a beautiful gold piece of thread lightly connected to the crown of your head extended to the sky. You want your joints to feel lightly stacked on one another. This will encourage you to engage your core muscles abdominals, obliques, and lower back. Avoid slouching and humping over. Keep the body at a peaceful attention throughout the day.

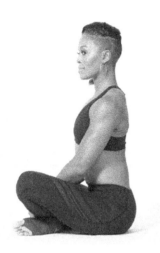

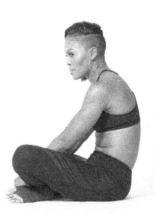

*Spine Lengthener Variation Posture Check*

69

# TWENTY-SIX

# Abdominal Stretch and Heart Opener (Cobra)

Start by lying down on the floor. Place your hands flush on the floor under your shoulders and outside of your torso. Inhale deeply. Exhale and press through your palms and slowly peel your body off of the floor leaving your hips and legs connected to the floor. Inhale deeply. Exhale and hold the stretch 20 seconds. Keep your neck extended and your chin level. Avoid slouching or sinking your head into your shoulders. Slowly lower your body back to the floor. Repeat stretch 3 times.

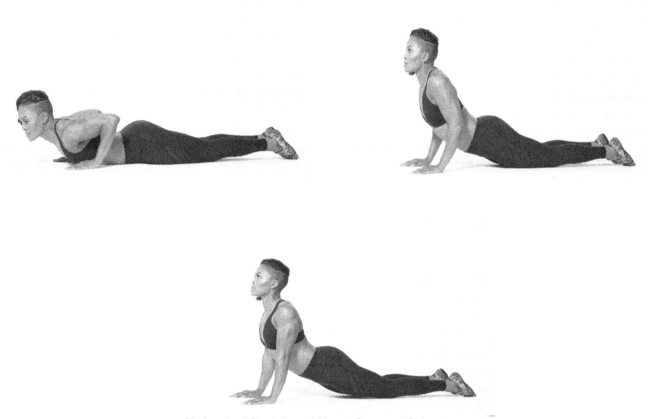

*Abdominal Stretch and Heart Opener (Cobra)*

# TWENTY-SEVEN

# Neck Roll Variation with Cobra

Start by lying down on the floor. Place your hands flush on the floor under your shoulders and outside of your torso. Inhale deeply. Exhale and press through your palms and slowly peel your body off of the floor leaving your hips and legs connected to the floor. Inhale deeply. Exhale and hold the stretch 20 seconds. Keep your neck extended and your chin level. Avoid slouching or sinking your head into your shoulders. Turn you head to the right. Inhale deeply. Exhale and slowly roll your head to the left. Repeat 3 times

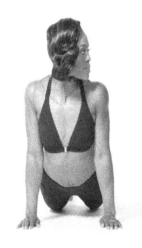
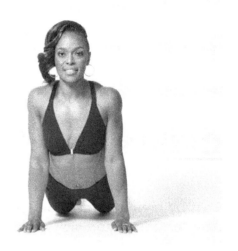

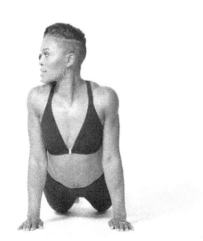
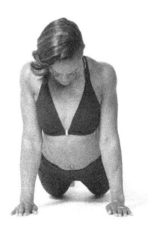

*Neck Roll Variation with Cobra*

# TWENTY-EIGHT

# Child's Pose Low Back Stretch

Start by laying on the floor face down with your with hands and knees on the floor. Inhale deeply. Exhale and slowly shift your hips back so your butt rests on your heels. Your hands stay flush on the floor and arms stretch out to reach in the opposite direction of the hips and butt. Inhale deeply. Exhale and relax deeper into the stretch. Hold 30 seconds.

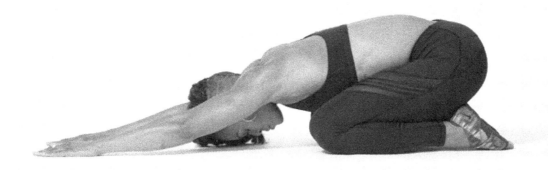

*Child's Pose Low Back Stretch*

# TWENTY-NINE

# Child's Pose Variation

Start by laying on the floor face down with your hands and knees on the floor. Inhale deeply. Exhale and slowly shift your hips back so your butt rests on your heels. Your hands stay flush on the floor and arms stretch out to reach the opposite direction of the hips and butt. Inhale deeply. Exhale and slide your arms next to your hips, turning your hands so your palms face the sky. Turn your head to the right. Hold 30 seconds. Turn your head to the left. Hold 30 seconds.

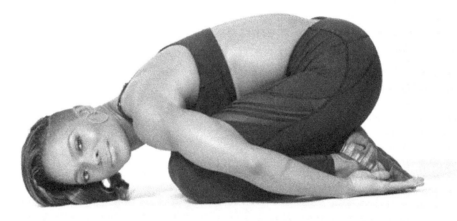

*Child's Pose Variation*

# THIRTY

# Chest and Shoulder Stretch (Heart Opener)

Start in a seated position. Open your arms out to the side pointing down at an angle. Open your hands and let your palms face forward. Inhale deeply. Exhale and open your arms wide. Keep your shoulders relaxed. Feel the energy release through your fingertips. Inhale deeply. Exhale and hold 30 seconds. Repeat 3 times.

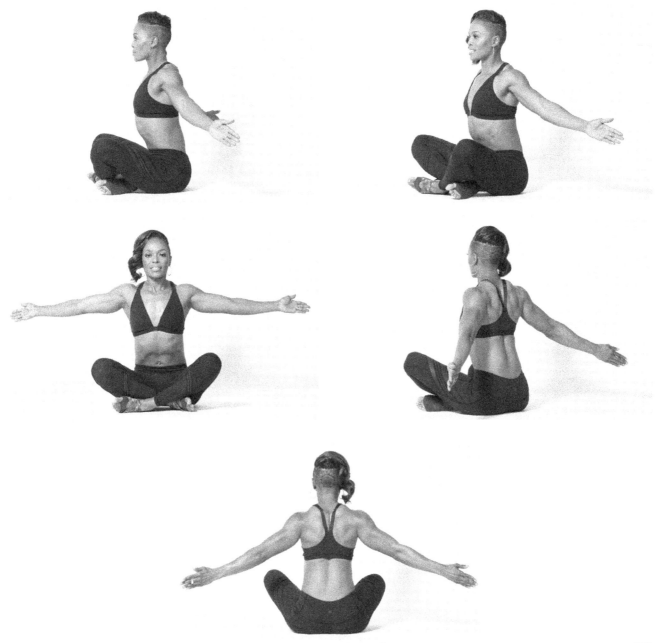

*Chest and Shoulder Stretch (Heart Opener)*

# THIRTY-ONE

# Chest Opener

Start in a seated position. Extend your arms out to the side and bend at the elbows with hands pointing towards the sky. Let your palms face forward. Inhale deeply. Exhale, opening your arms wide yet keep the bend in the elbow. Inhale deeply. Exhale and hold for 20 seconds. Repeat 3 times.

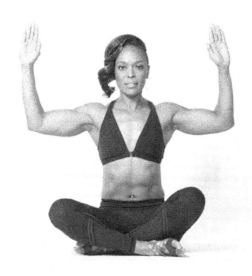

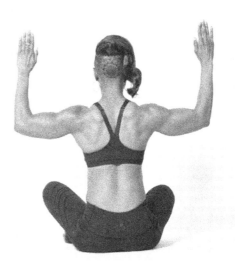

*Chest Opener*

# THIRTY-TWO

## Standing Full Body Stretch

Begin this stretch standing. Extend your arms up to the sky. Inhale deeply. Exhale and feel the stretch from the base of your body, the soles of your feet, through your legs, your hips, torso, in and through your arms to your fingertips. Inhale deeply. Exhale and continue to stretch staying rooted to the ground yet lifted in the core. Hold 30 seconds. Relax and bring arms down. Repeat 3 times.

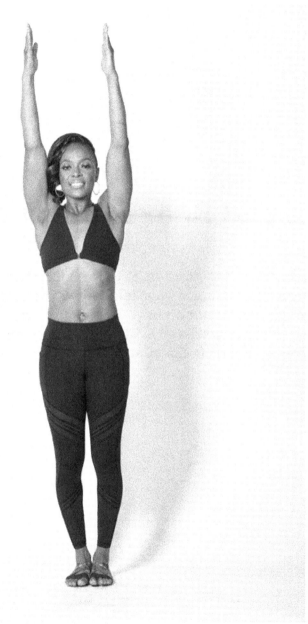

*Standing Full Body Stretch*

# THIRTY-THREE

# Shoulder and Rear Deltoid

Begin this stretch in a standing position. Extend your right arm in front of you. Slowly take the right arm across your body. Place your left hand on your right arm between the elbow and the wrist. Firmly hold the right arm in your left hand. Inhale deeply. As you exhale, gently pull the right arm closer to your body. Keep your right shoulder down and away from your chin. Hold 15 seconds. Switch to the other arm. Repeat stretch on both arms 2 times.

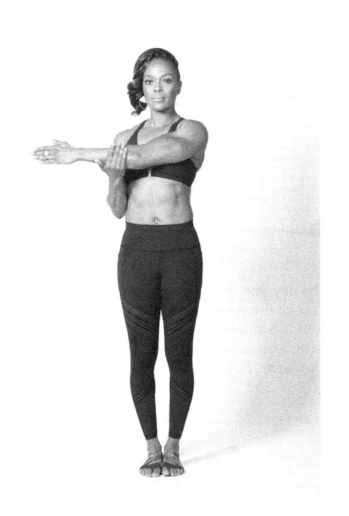

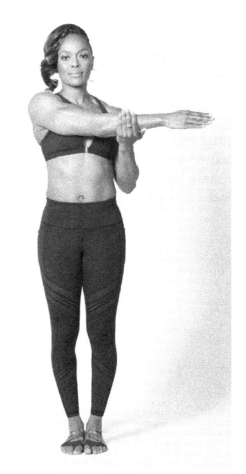

*Shoulder and Rear Deltoid Stretch*

# THIRTY-FOUR

# Standing Tricep Stretch

Stand comfortably and stretch both arms up to the sky with energy extending through your fingertips. Bend the right arm at the elbow and reach for your left shoulder with your right hand. Reach your left arm up and over placing your left hand on the side of your right elbow. Inhale deeply. As you exhale, gently place pressure on your right arm with you left hand. Hold this stretch for 15 seconds. Switch to the other arm. Repeat 2 times.

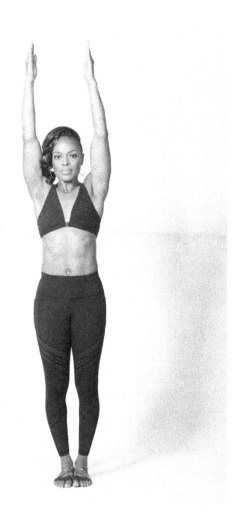

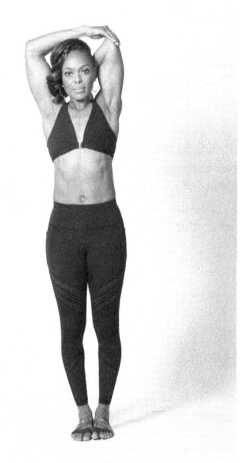

*Standing Tricep Stretch*

# THIRTY-FIVE

# Standing Chest Opener Shoulder Stretch Variation

Stand comfortably. Open your arms out to the side pointing down at an angle. Open your hands and let your palms face forward. Inhale deeply. Exhale and open your arms wide. Keep your shoulders relaxed. Bring your hands close to each other behind you until your fingertips touch. Interlace your fingers. Feel energy through the front of your shoulder and your chest. Inhale deeply. Exhale and hold 30 seconds. Repeat 3 times.

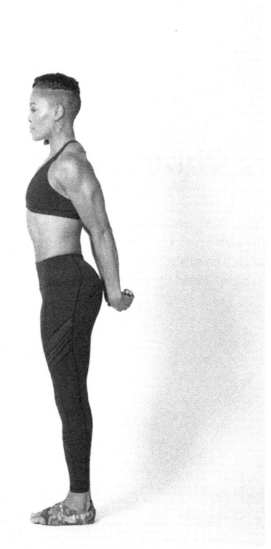

*Standing Chest Opener Shoulder Chest Variation*

# THIRTY-SIX

# Standing Oblique Stretch

Stand comfortably. Place your left arm down by your side. Allow you palm to rest on your leg. Extend your right arm up to the sky. Inhale deeply. Exhale and lean over to your left. Stretch your arm in an arch like motion. Inhale deeply. Exhale and gently bend a little more without collapsing in the side. Hold 20 seconds. Relax right arm down. Repeat on the other side.

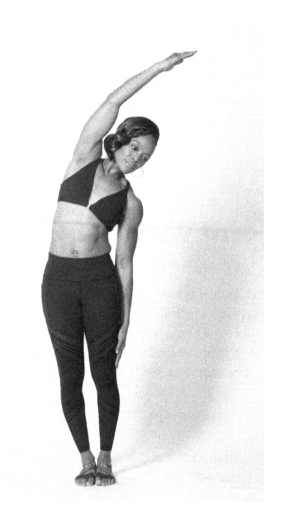
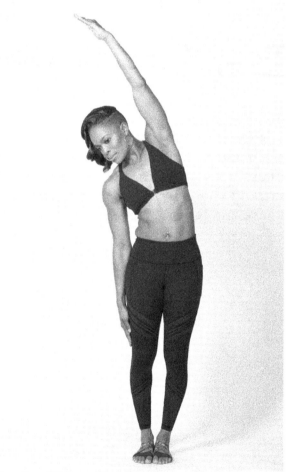

*Standing Oblique Stretch*

91

# THIRTY-SEVEN

# Body Warm Up Flow – Joint Warm Up

Stand with legs wider than shoulder width. Bend at the waist as if you are reaching down to wipe dust off a coffee table with both hands and two cloths. Imagine you are wiping this table and making an infinity sign design on the table. As you visualize this design, let your entire body participate. Bend your knees, move your hips, and glide side to side while you're moving your hands. Inhale deeply. Exhale and continue this rhythmic flow for 30 seconds. Pause and repeat 2 times.

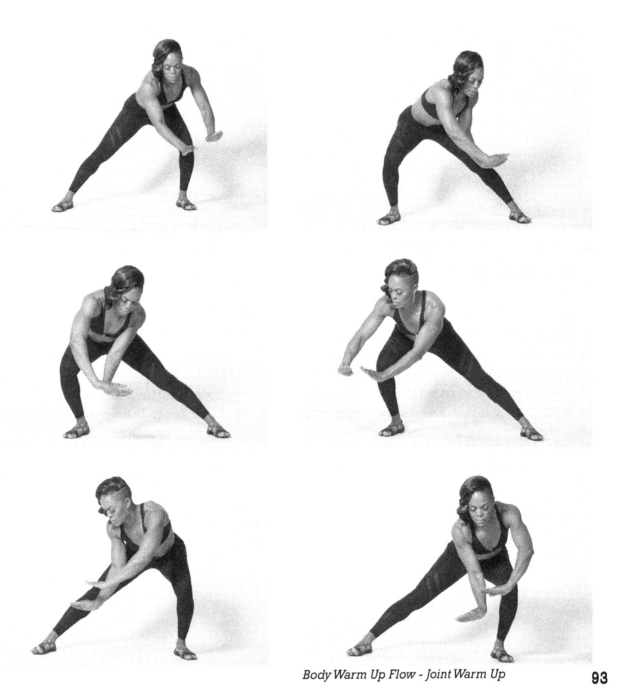

*Body Warm Up Flow - Joint Warm Up*

# THIRTY-EIGHT

# Hamstring Low Back Stretch Advanced Variation

Stand comfortably. Inhale deeply. Exhale and slowly hinge at the hips, lowering your upper body to the floor while keeping your legs straight. Once you are at your lowest level gently place your palms behind your ankles or your calves. Inhale deeply. Exhale slowly, placing your palms or fingertips on the floor. Inhale deeply. Exhale bending the knees and lowering your butt to your heels, keeping the gaze of your eyes to the floor. Inhale deeply. Exhale and lift the hips back to the ceiling and lower 7 times, keeping your hands or fingertips connected to the floor. Inhale deeply. Exhale and bring your right heel off the floor. Place the right heel back on the floor. Then lift the left heel off the floor. Place it back down. Repeat 7 times.

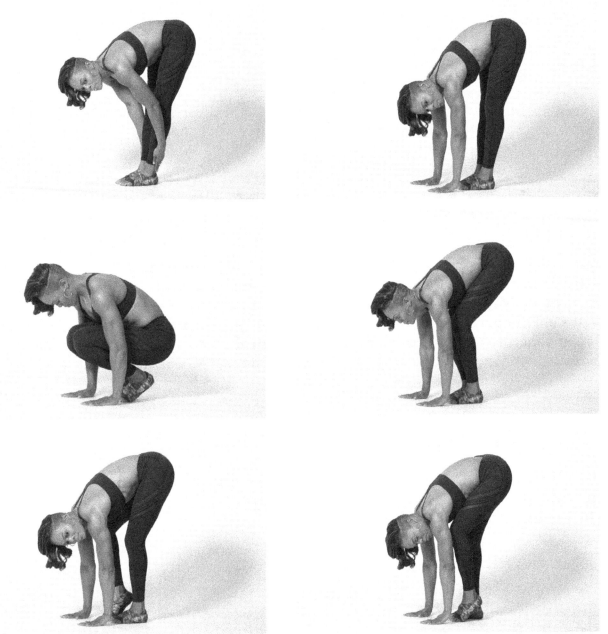

*Hamstring Low Back Stretch Advanced Variation*   **95**

# THIRTY-NINE

# Standing Quad Stretch Variation

Stand comfortably. Stretch your right arm to the sky. To maintain better balance you can extend your arm out in front of you and hold at shoulder level. Inhale deeply. Exhale and slowly bend your left leg at the knee. Extend your left arm back and gently hold your left leg at the ankle, pant leg, or heel of shoe. Inhale deeply. Exhale and continue to firmly hold your leg in bent. Keep your knees side by side. Do not allow the leg to open out to the side or the body to lean forward. Hold for 20 to 25 seconds. Repeat on both legs 2 times.

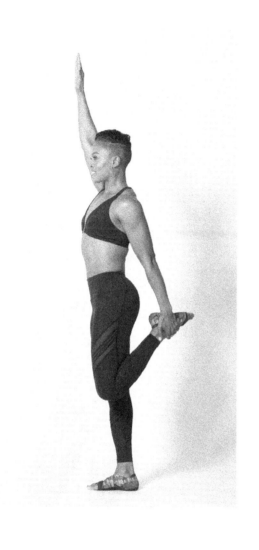

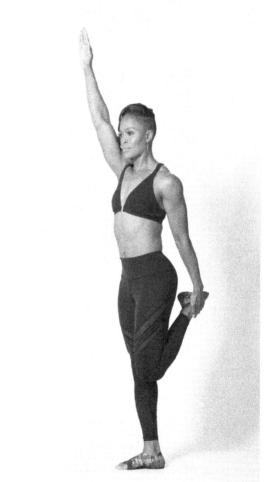

*Standing Quad Stretch Variation*

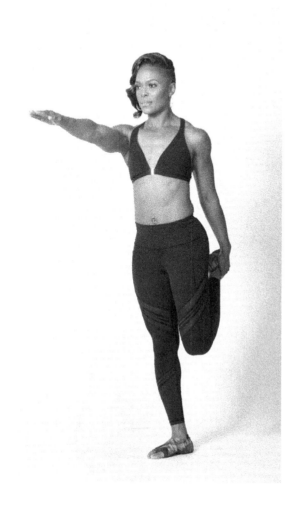

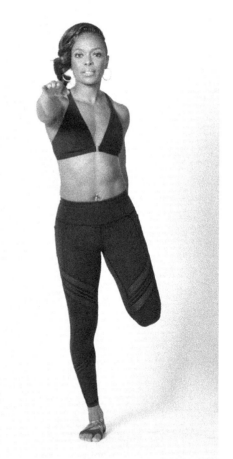

*Standing Quad Stretch Variation*

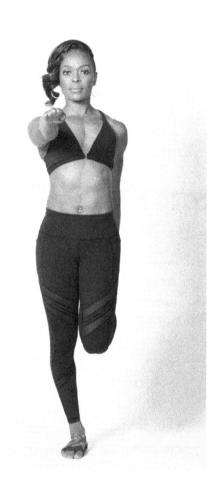

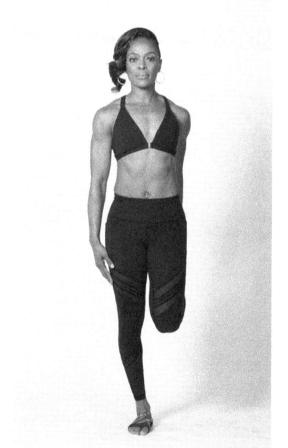

*Standing Quad Stretch Variation*

# FORTY

# Standing Hamstring Stretch Variation

Stand comfortably. Extend your right leg out and lower your hips down and back.  Inhale deeply.  Exhale and reach both hands out toward your right foot. Inhale deeply.  Exhale and stretch your hands down closer to your shin, ankle, foot, or toes.  Flex and point your toes away and toward the floor. Hold 20 seconds.  Repeat both legs 2 times.

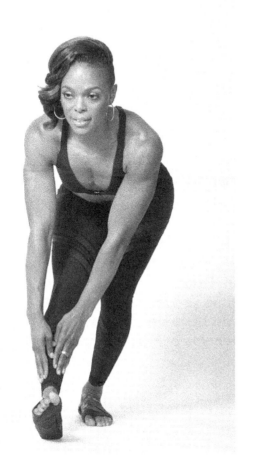

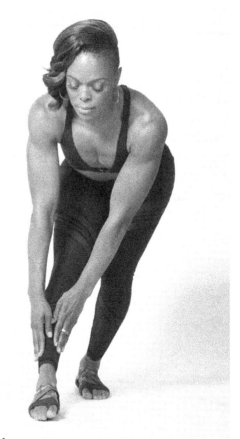

*Standing Hamstring Stretch Variation*

# FORTY-ONE

# Dynamic Stretching Front Leg Raises

Stand comfortably. Extend both arms up toward the sky creating the letter Y with your body. Inhale deeply. Exhale and raise your left leg hip level and lower your right arm to shoulder level. Inhale return arm and leg to starting point. Exhale and raise your right leg hip level and lower your left arm to shoulder level. Each time you reach out your arm stretch forward and lengthen your upper body. This stretching can be done standing in place or in motion. If you have enough space to move with this stretch you can walk forward for 30 movements total. 15 on each side.

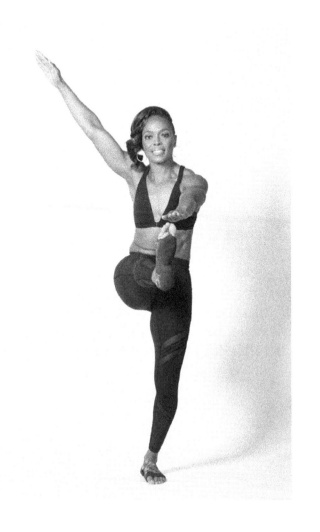
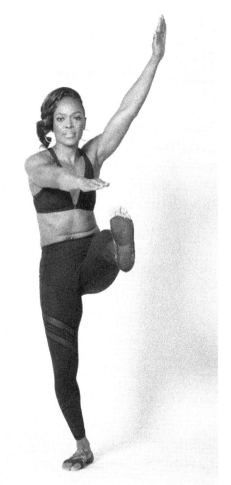

*Dynamic Stretching Front Leg Raises*

# FORTY-TWO

# Standing Hip Flexor Variation

Stand comfortably. Extend your left leg behind you with your right toes touching the ground while keeping your heel lifted. Inhale deeply. Exhale and lower your heel of your left leg and bend the knee of your right leg. Inhale deeply. Exhale and hold stretch 20 to 25 seconds. Inhale deeply lower left knee and hold 10 seconds with left heel off the floor. Repeat on both sides 2 times.

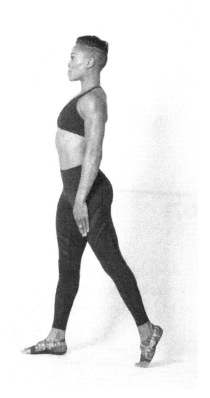

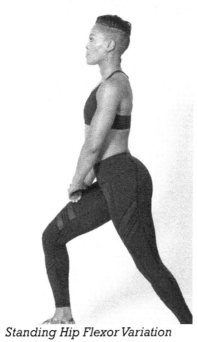

*Standing Hip Flexor Variation*

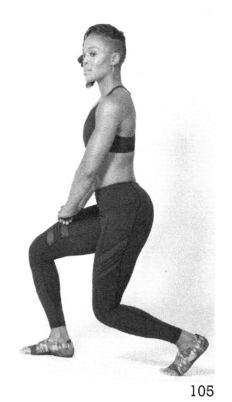

# FORTY-THREE

# Kneeling Quad Stretch Variation

Start kneeling on left knee. Place right foot flat on the floor. Inhale deeply. Exhale and reach back toward your left leg lifting your left foot off the floor. Gently grab your left leg at the ankle, pant leg, or heel of your shoe. Inhale deeply. Exhale and hold for 20 seconds. Switch to other leg and repeat.

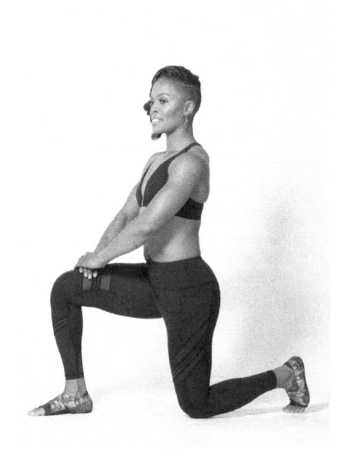

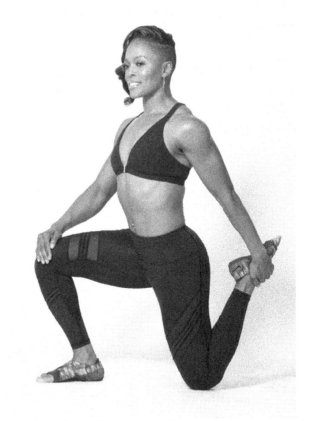

*Kneeling Quad Stretch Variation*

# FORTY-FOUR

# Hip Flexor Stretch

Start kneeling on left knee.   Place right foot flat on the floor.  Extend both arms up to the sky. Inhale deeply. Exhale and slowly lean back at the hip and feel a small contraction in the lower back muscles. Inhale deeply. Hold the gentle stretch for 30 seconds. Repeat on both sides 2 times.

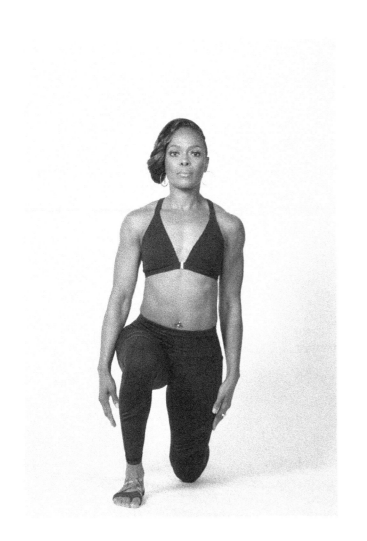

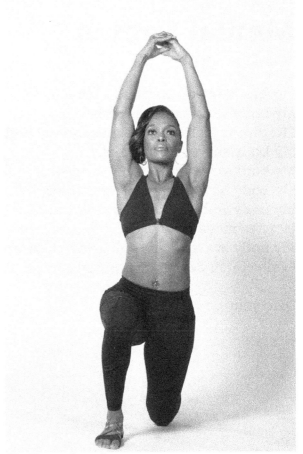

*Hip Flexor Stretch*

# FORTY-FIVE

# Mental Stretch

I love, accept, respect and appreciate my body.
My body serves me perfectly.
I forgive myself for disrespecting my body in any way.
My body serves me perfectly.
My body is my most valuable asset.
My body has unlimited possibilities.
My body will do whatever I tell it to do.
I love to move it.
My body is a gift and I will love it more and more each day.
I will stretch beyond my mental and physical boundaries.

Love your body.

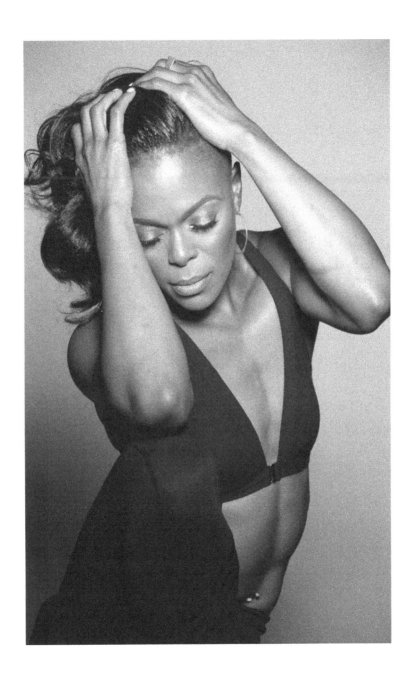

CPSIA information can be obtained
at www.ICGtesting.com
Printed in the USA
BVHW061928030320
573705BV00005B/10